The Ultimate Keto

CW00520723

for Carb Lovers

The Latest Collection of Mouthwatering

Recipes To Lose Weight, Increase Energy And

Boost Your Immune System.

Virginia Castro

© Copyright 2021 by Virginia Castro

- All rights reserved.

The following Book is reproduced below with the goal of providing information that is as accurate and reliable as possible. Regardless, purchasing this Book can be seen as consent to the fact that both the publisher and the author of this book are in no way experts on the topics discussed within and that any recommendations or suggestions that are made herein are for entertainment purposes only. Professionals should be consulted as needed prior to undertaking any of the action endorsed herein.

This declaration is deemed fair and valid by both the American Bar Association and the Committee of Publishers Association and is legally binding throughout the United States.

Furthermore, the transmission, duplication, or reproduction of any of the following work including specific information will be considered an illegal act irrespective of if it is done electronically or in print. This extends to creating a secondary or tertiary copy of the work or a recorded copy and is only allowed with the express written consent from the Publisher. All additional right reserved.

The information in the following pages is broadly considered a truthful and accurate account of facts and as such, any inattention, use, or misuse of the information in question by the reader will render any resulting actions solely under their purview. There are no scenarios in which the publisher or the original author of this work can be in any fashion deemed liable for any hardship or damages that may befall them after undertaking information described herein.

Additionally, the information in the following pages is intended only for informational purposes and should thus be thought of as universal. As befitting its nature, it is presented without assurance regarding its prolonged validity or interim quality. Trademarks that are mentioned are done without written consent and can in no way be considered an endorsement from the trademark holder.

Table of Contents

POULTRY RECIPES

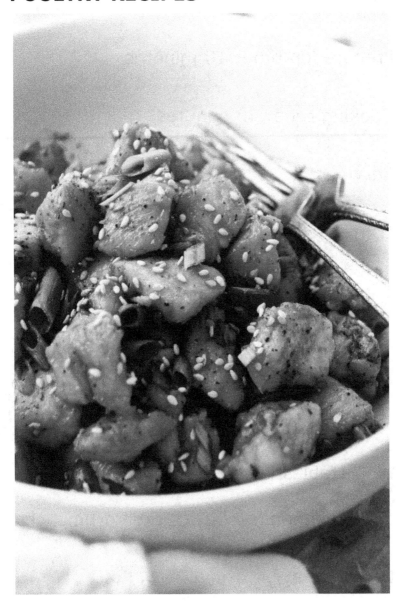

1. Thyme Roasted Drumsticks

Preparation time: 10 minutes

Cooking time: 40 minutes

Servings: 2

Ingredients:

- 1stick unsalted butter, softened

- 4 cloves garlic, minced

- Sea salt and ground black pepper, to taste

- 1tablespoon fresh thyme leaves

- 2pounds (907 g) chicken drumsticks

Directions:

1. In a mixing bowl, thoroughly combine the butter, garlic, salt, black

pepper, and thyme. Rub this mixture all over the chicken drumsticks.

2. Lay the chicken drumsticks on a parchment-lined baking tray. Bake in the preheated oven at 390ºF (199ºC) until an instant-read thermometer reads 165ºF (74ºC) about 40 minutes.

3. Place under the preheated broiler for 1to 2minutes if you'd like the golden, crisp skin. Bon appétit!

Nutrition: calorie

s: 342 fat: 24.3g protein: 28.1g carbs:

1.7g net carbs: 1.4g fiber: 0.3g

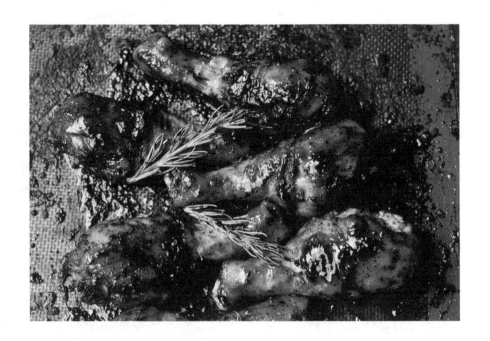

2. Rice Wine Duck with White Onion

Preparation time: 5 minutes

Cooking time: 25 minutes

Servings: 2

Ingredients:

- 1½ pounds (680 g) duck breast

  1tablespoon sesame oil

- 1white onion, chopped

- ¼ cup rice wine

- 3 teaspoons soy sauce

Directions:

1. Gently score the duck breast skin in a tight crosshatch pattern using a sharp knife.

2. Heat the sesame oil in a skillet over moderate heat. Now, sauté the onion until tender and translucent.

3. Add in the duck breasts; sear the duck breasts for 10 to 13 minutes or until the skin looks crispy with golden brown color; drain off the duck fat from the skillet.

4. Flip the breasts over and sear the other side for 3 minutes. Deglaze the skillet with rice wine, scraping up any

brown bits stuck to the bottom. Transfer to a baking pan; add the rice wine and soy sauce to the baking pan.

5. Roast in the preheated oven at 400ºF (205ºC) for 4 minutes for medium-rare (145ºF / 63ºC), or 6 minutes for medium (165ºF / 74ºC).

6. Serve garnished with sesame seeds if desired. Enjoy!

Nutrition: calories: 264   fat: 11.4g

protein: 34.2g   carbs: 3.6g   net carbs:

3.0g fiber: 0.6g

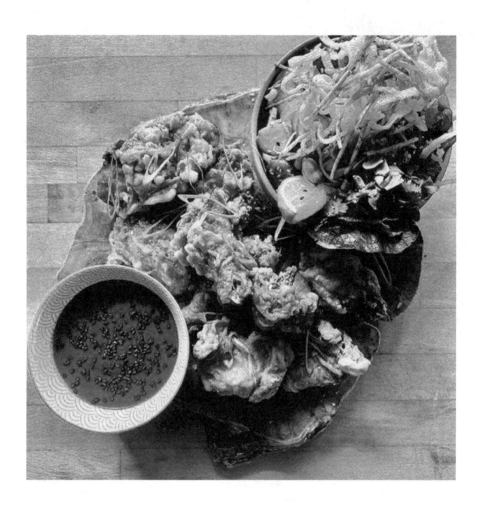

3. Bacon and Chicken Frittata

Preparation time: 15 minutes

Cooking time: 25 minutes

Servings: 2

Ingredients:

- 4 slices of bacon
- 1pound (454 g) chicken breasts, cut into small strips
- 1red bell pepper, chopped
- 1onion, chopped
- 2garlic cloves, minced
- eggs
- ½ cup yogurt
- ½ teaspoon hot paprika

- Sea salt and freshly ground black pepper
- ½ teaspoon oregano
- ½ teaspoon rosemary
- 1cup Asiago cheese, shredded

Directions:

1. In an oven-safe pan, cook the bacon until crisp, crumbling with a fork; reserve. Then, in the same pan, cook the chicken breasts for 5 to 6 minutes or until no longer pink; reserve.

2. Then, sauté the pepper, onion, and garlic in the bacon grease. Cook until they have softened.

3. In a mixing bowl, whisk the eggs with the yogurt, paprika, salt, black pepper, oregano, and rosemary. Add the bacon and chicken back to the pan.

4. Pour the egg mixture over the chicken mixture. Top with Asiago cheese. Bake in the preheated oven at 390°F (199°C) for 20 minutes until the eggs are puffed and opaque.

5. You can cut a slit in the center of the frittata to check the doneness. Bon appétit!

Nutrition: calories: 485   fat: 31.7g protein: 41.8g   carbs: 5.7g   net carbs: 4.9g fiber: 0.8g

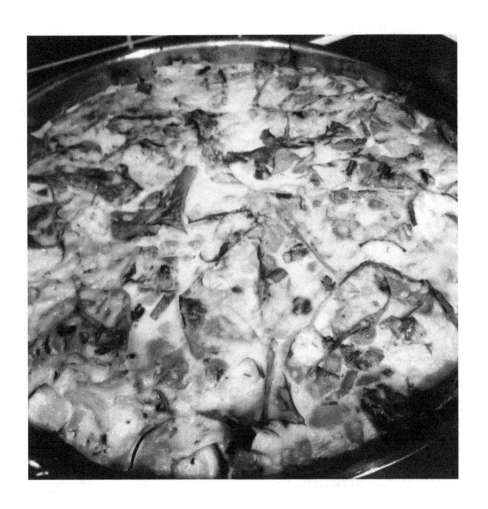

4.　Mediterranean Roasted Chicken Drumettes

Preparation time: 15 minutes

Cooking time: 20 minutes

Servings: 2

Ingredients:

- 2tablespoons olive oil
- 1½ pounds (680 g) chicken drumettes
- 2cloves garlic, minced
- 1thyme sprig
- 1rosemary sprig
- ½ teaspoon dried oregano

- Sea salt and freshly ground black pepper, to taste
- 2tablespoons Greek cooking wine
- ½ cup chicken bone broth
- 1red onion, cut into wedges
- 2bell peppers, sliced

Directions:

1. Start by preheating your oven to 420ºF (216ºC). Brush the sides and bottom a baking dish with 1tablespoon of olive oil.

2. Heat the remaining tablespoon of olive oil in a saucepan over a moderate flame. Brown the chicken drumettes for 5 to 6 minutes per side.

3. Transfer the warm chicken drumettes to a baking dish. Add the garlic, spices, wine and broth. Scatter red onion and peppers around chicken drumettes.

4. Roast in the preheated oven for about 13 minutes. Serve immediately and enjoy!

Nutrition: calories: 219   fat: 9.2g

protein: 28.5g   carbs: 4.2g   net carbs:

3.5g fiber: 0.7g

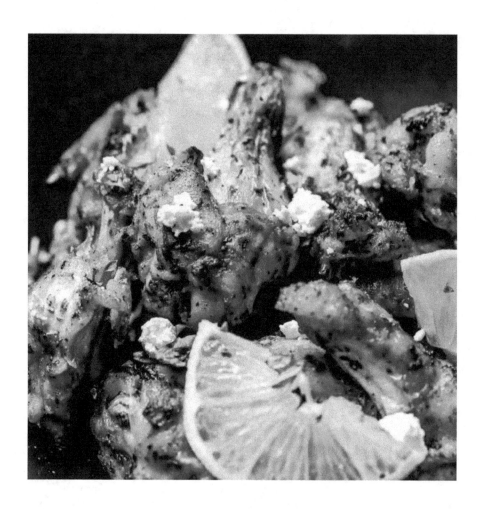

5. Mediterranean Chicken with Peppers and Olives

Preparation time: 15 minutes

Cooking time: 15 minutes

Servings: 2

Ingredients:

- 2chicken drumsticks, boneless and skinless
- 1tablespoon extra-virgin olive oil
- Sea salt and ground black pepper, to season
- 2bell peppers, deveined and halved
- 1small chili pepper, finely chopped
- 2tablespoons Greek aioli

- Kalamata olives, pitted

Directions:

1. Brush the chicken drumsticks with the olive oil. Season the chicken drumsticks with salt and black pepper.

2. Preheat your grill to moderate heat. Grill the chicken drumsticks for 8 minutes; turn them over and add the bell peppers.

3. Grill them for a further 5 minutes. Transfer to a serving platter; top with chopped chili pepper and Greek aioli.

4. Garnish with Kalamata olives and serve warm. Enjoy!

Nutrition: calories: 400   fat: 31.3g protein: 24.5g   carbs: 5.0g   net carbs: 3.9g fiber: 1.1g

6.   Chicken Puttanesca

Preparation time: 15 minutes

Cooking time: 20 minutes

Servings: 2

Ingredients:

- 2tablespoons olive oil

- 1bell pepper, chopped

- 1red onion, chopped

- 1teaspoon garlic, minced

- 1½ pounds (680 g) chicken wings, boneless

- 2cups tomato sauce

- 1tablespoon capers

- ¼ teaspoon red pepper, crushed

- ¼ cup Parmesan cheese, preferably freshly grated

- 2basil sprigs, chopped

Directions:

1. Heat the olive oil in a non-stick skillet over a moderate flame. Once hot, sauté the bell peppers and onions until tender and fragrant.

2. Stir in the garlic and continue to cook an additional 30 seconds.

3. Stir in the chicken wings, tomato sauce, capers, and red pepper; continue to cook for a further 20 minutes or until everything is heated through.

4. Serve garnished with freshly grated Parmesan and basil. Bon appétit!

Nutrition: calories: 266   fat: 11.3g protein: 32.6g   carbs: 6.4g   net carbs: 5.1g fiber: 1.3g

7.   Italian Parmesan Turkey Fillets

Preparation time: 10 minutes

Cooking time: 15 minutes

Servings: 2

Ingredients:

- 2eggs

- 1cup sour cream

- 1teaspoon Italian seasoning blend

- Kosher salt and ground black pepper, to taste

- ½ cup grated Parmesan cheese

- 2pounds (907 g) turkey fillets

Directions:

1. In a mixing bowl, whisk the eggs until frothy and light. Stir in the sour cream and continue whisking until well combined.

2. In another bowl, mix the Italian seasoning blend with the salt, black pepper, and Parmesan cheese; mix to combine well.

3. Dip the turkey fillets into the egg mixture; then, press them into the Parmesan mixture.

4. Cook in the greased frying pan until browned on all sides. Bon appétit!

Nutrition: calories: 336   fat: 12.7g
protein: 47.5g   carbs: 5.2g   net carbs:
5.0g fiber: 0.2g

8.   Veg Stuffed Chicken with Spiralized Cucumber

Preparation time: 20 minutes

Cooking time: 55 minutes

Servings: 2

Ingredients:

Chicken:

- 2tablespoons butter
- 4 chicken breasts
- 1cup baby spinach
- 1carrot, shredded
- 1tomato, chopped
- ¼ cup goat cheese
- Salt and black pepper, to taste

- 1teaspoon dried oregano

Salad:

- 2cucumbers, spiralized
- 2tablespoons olive oil
- 1tablespoon rice vinegar

Directions:

1. Preheat oven to 390ºF (199ºC) and grease a baking dish with cooking spray.

2. Place a pan over medium heat. Melt half of the butter and sauté spinach, carrot, and tomato until tender, for about 5 minutes. Season with salt

and pepper. Transfer to a medium bowl and let cool for 10 minutes.

3. Add in the goat cheese and oregano, stir and set to one side. Cut the chicken breasts lengthwise and stuff with the cheese mixture and set into the baking dish.

4. On top, put the remaining butter and bake until cooked through for 20-30 minutes.

5. Arrange the cucumbers on a serving platter, season with salt, black pepper, olive oil, and vinegar. Top with the chicken and pour over the sauce.

Nutrition: calories: 618   fat: 46.4g

protein: 40.6g   carbs: 9.4g   net carbs:

7.6g fiber: 1.8g

FISH AND SEAFOOD RECIPES

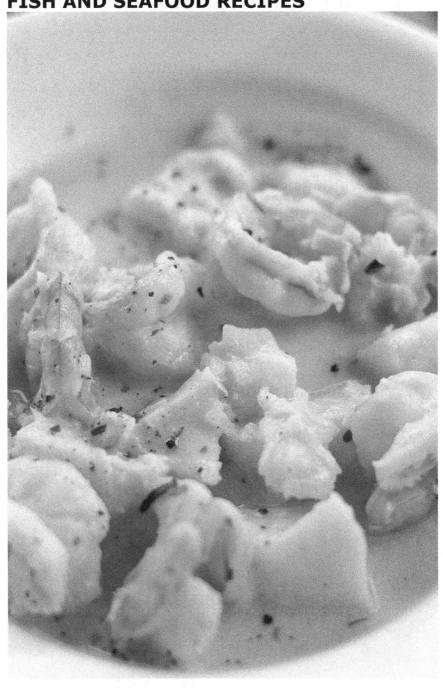

9.   Dijon-Tarragon Salmon

Preparation time:10 minutes

Cooking time: 10 minutes

Servings: 2

Ingredients:

- 4 salmon fillets

- ¾ teaspoon fresh thyme

- 1tablespoon butter

- ¾ teaspoon tarragon

- Salt and black pepper to taste

Sauce:

- ¼ cup Dijon mustard

- 2tablespoons white wine

- ½ teaspoon tarragon

- ¼ cup heavy cream

Directions:

1. Season the salmon with thyme, tarragon, salt, and black pepper. Melt the butter in a pan over medium heat. Add salmon and cook for about 4-5 minutes on both sides until the salmon is cooked through. Remove to a warm dish and cover.

2. To the same pan, add the sauce ingredients over low heat and simmer until the sauce is slightly thickened, stirring continually. Cook for 60 seconds to infuse the flavors

and adjust the seasoning. Serve the salmon, topped with the sauce.

Nutrition: calories: 538 fat: 26.5g protein: 66.9g carbs: 2.1g net carbs: 1.4g fiber: 0.7g

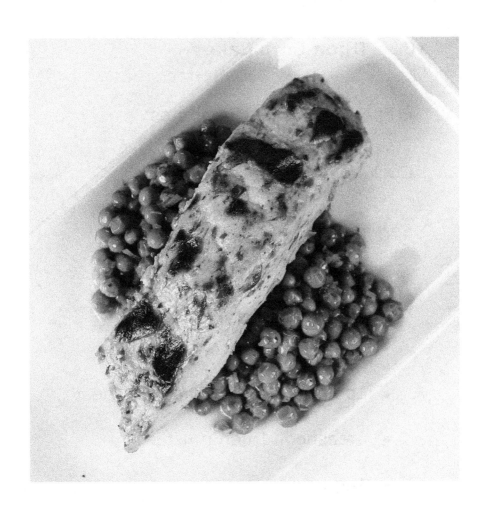

10. Dijon Crab Cakes

Preparation time: 10 minutes

Cooking time: 5 minutes

Servings: 2

Ingredients:

- 1tablespoon coconut oil
- 1pound (454 g) lump crab meat
- 1teaspoon Dijon mustard
- 1egg
- ¼ cup mayonnaise
- 1tablespoon coconut flour
- 1tablespoon cilantro, chopped

Directions:

1. In a bowl, add crab meat, mustard, mayonnaise, coconut flour, egg, cilantro, salt, and pepper; mix to combine. Make patties out of the mixture. Melt coconut oil in a skillet over medium heat. Add crab patties and cook for 2-3 minutes per side. Remove to kitchen paper.

2. Serve.

Nutrition: calories: 316 fat: 24.3g protein: 15.2g carbs: 1.8g net carbs: 1.5g fiber: 0.3g

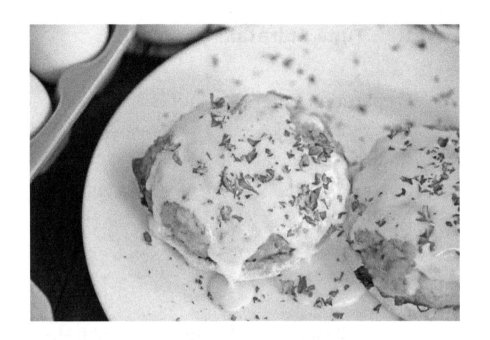

11.   Tuna Shirataki Pad Thai

Preparation time:15 minutes

Cooking time: 5 minutes

Servings: 2

Ingredients:

- 1(7-ounce / 198-g) pack shirataki noodles
- 4 cups water
- 1red bell pepper, sliced
- 2tablespoons soy sauce, sugar-free
- 1tablespoon ginger-garlic paste
- 1teaspoon chili powder
- 1tablespoon water
- 4 tuna steaks

- Salt and black pepper to taste

- 1tablespoon olive oil

- 1tablespoon parsley, chopped

Directions:

1. In a colander, rinse the shirataki noodles with running cold water. Bring a pot of salted water to a boil; blanch the noodles for 2minutes. Drain and set aside.

2. Preheat a grill on medium-high. Season the tuna with salt and black pepper, brush with olive oil, and grill covered. Cook for 3 minutes on each side.

3. In a bowl, whisk soy sauce, ginger-garlic paste, olive oil, chili powder, and water. Add bell pepper, and noodles and toss to coat. Assemble noodles and tuna in serving plate and garnish with parsley.

Nutrition: calories: 288 fat: 16.1g protein: 23.2g carbs: 7.7g net carbs: 6.7g fiber: 1.0g

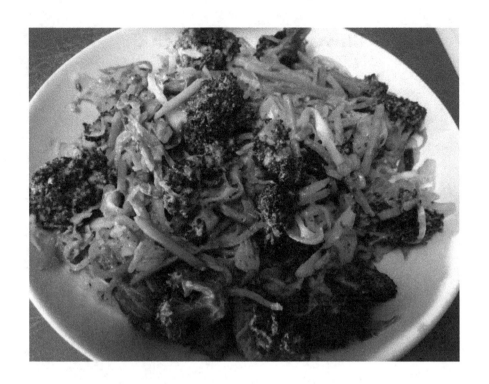

12. Chive-Sauced Chili Cod

Preparation time: 10 minutes

Cooking time: 20 minutes

Servings: 2

Ingredients:

- 1teaspoon chili powder
- 4 cod fillets
- Salt and black pepper to taste
- 1tablespoon olive oil
- 1garlic clove, minced
- 1/3 cup lemon juice
- 2tablespoons vegetable stock
- 2tablespoons chives, chopped

Directions:

1. Preheat oven to 400°F (205°C) and grease a baking dish with cooking spray. Rub the cod fillets with chili powder, salt, and pepper and lay in the dish. Bake for 10-15 minutes.

2. In a skillet over low heat, warm olive oil and sauté garlic for 1minute. Add lemon juice, vegetable stock, and chives. Season with salt, pepper, and cook for 3 minutes until the stock slightly reduces. Divide fish into 2plates, top with sauce, and serve.

Nutrition: calories: 450 fat: 35.2g protein: 20.1g carbs: 7.0g net carbs: 6.4g fiber: 0.6g

13.   Catalan Shrimp

Preparation time: 5 minutes

Cooking time: 20 minutes

Servings: 2

Ingredients:

- ¼ cup olive oil, divided
- 1pound (454 g) shrimp, deveined
- Salt to taste
- ¼ teaspoon cayenne pepper
- 3 garlic cloves, sliced
- 2tablespoons chopped parsley

Directions:

1. Warm olive oil in a large skillet over medium heat. Reduce the heat and

add the garlic; cook for 6-8 minutes, but make sure it doesn't brown or burn. Add the shrimp, season with salt and cayenne pepper, stir for one minute and turn off the heat. Let the shrimp finish cooking with the heat of the hot oil for about 8-10 minutes. Serve garnished with parsley.

Nutrition: calories: 442 fat: 28.9g protein: 43.2g carbs: 1.2g net carbs: 1.1g fiber: 0.1g

14.   Almond Breaded Hoki

Preparation time:15 minutes

Cooking time: 25 minutes

Servings: 2

Ingredients:

- 1cup flaked smoked hoki, bones removed
- 1cup cubed hoki fillets, cubed
- 4 eggs
- 1cup water
- 3 tablespoons almond flour
- 1onion, sliced
- 2cups sour cream
- 1tablespoon chopped parsley

- 1cup pork rinds, crushed

- 1cup grated Cheddar cheese

- Salt and black pepper to taste

- 2tablespoons butter

Directions:

1. Preheat the oven to 360ºF (182ºC) and lightly grease a baking dish with cooking spray.

2. Then, boil the eggs in water in a pot over medium heat to be well done for 10 minutes, run the eggs under cold

water and peel the shells. After, place on a cutting board and chop them.

3. Melt the butter in a saucepan over medium heat and sauté the onion for 4 minutes. Turn the heat off and stir in the almond flour to form a roux. Turn the heat back on and cook the roux to be golden brown and stir in the cream until the mixture is smooth. Season with salt and black pepper, and stir in the parsley.

4. Spread the smoked and cubed fish in the baking dish, sprinkle the eggs on top, and spoon the sauce over. In a bowl, mix the pork rinds with the

Cheddar cheese, and sprinkle it over the sauce.

5. Bake the casserole in the oven for 20 minutes until the top is golden and the sauce and cheese are bubbly. Remove the bake after and serve with a steamed green vegetable mix.

Nutrition: calories: 384 fat: 27.1g protein: 28.4g carbs: 3.9g net carbs: 3.6g fiber: 0.3g

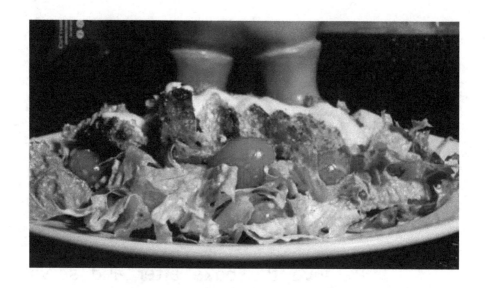

15.   Tuna Omelet Wraps

Preparation time:10 minutes

Cooking time: 10 minutes

Servings: 2

Ingredients:

- 1avocado, sliced

- 1tablespoon chopped chives

- 1cup canned tuna, drained

- 2spring onions, sliced

- 8 eggs, beaten

- 4 tablespoons mascarpone cheese

- 1tablespoon butter

- Salt and black pepper, to taste

Directions:

1. In a small bowl, combine the chives and mascarpone cheese; set aside. Melt the butter in a pan over medium heat. Add the eggs to the pan and cook for about 3 minutes. Flip the omelet over and continue cooking for another 2minutes until golden. Season with salt and black pepper.

2. Remove the omelet to a plate and spread the chive mixture over. Arrange the tuna, avocado, and onion slices. Wrap the omelet and serve immediately.

Nutrition: calories: 480 fat: 37.8g protein: 26.8g carbs: 9.9g net carbs: 6.3g fiber: 3.6g

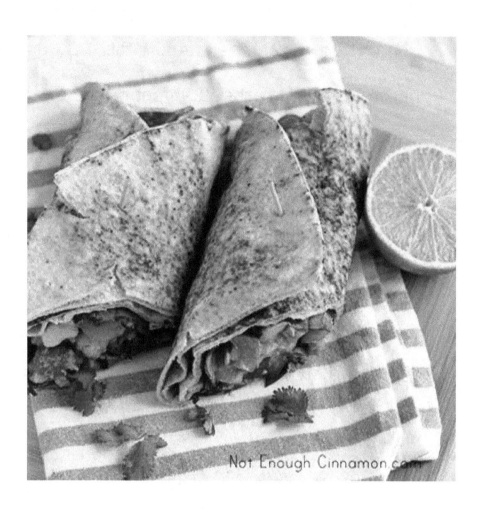

Not Enough Cinnamon.com

16. Seared Scallops with Sausage

Preparation time: 10 minutes

Cooking time: 10 minutes

Servings: 2

Ingredients:

- 2tablespoons butter

- 12fresh scallops, rinsed

- 8 ounces (227 g) sausage, chopped

- 1red bell pepper, sliced

- 1red onion, finely chopped

- 1cup Grana Padano, grated

- Salt and black pepper to taste

Directions:

1. Melt half of the butter in a skillet over medium heat, and cook the onion and bell pepper for 5 minutes until tender. Add the sausage and stir-fry for another 5 minutes. Remove and set aside.

2. Pat dry scallops with paper towels, and season with salt and pepper. Add the remaining butter to the skillet and sear scallops for 2minutes on each side to have a golden brown color. Add the sausage mixture back, and warm through. Transfer to

serving platter and top with Grana Padano cheese.

Nutrition: calories: 835 fat: 61.9g protein: 55.9g carbs: 10.5g net carbs: 9.4g fiber: 1.1g

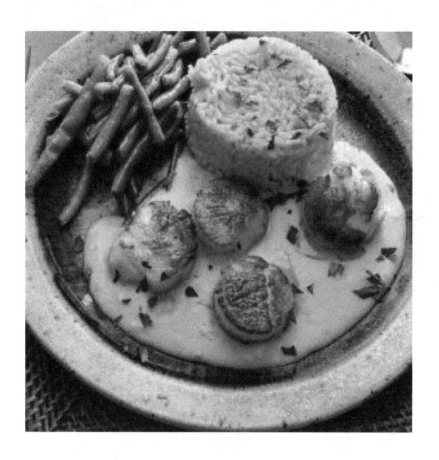

17. Baked Tilapia with Black Olives

Preparation time:15 minutes

Cooking time: 25 minutes

Servings: 2

Ingredients:

- 4 tilapia fillets

- 2garlic cloves, minced

- 1teaspoon basil, chopped

- 1cup canned tomatoes

- ¼ tablespoon chili powder

- 2tablespoons white wine

- 1tablespoon olive oil

- ½ red onion, chopped

- 2tablespoons parsley

- 10 black olives, pitted and halved

Directions:

1. Preheat oven to 350ºF (180ºC).

2. Heat the olive oil in a skillet over medium heat and cook the onion and garlic for about 3 minutes. Stir in tomatoes, olives, chili powder, and white wine and bring the mixture to a boil. Reduce the heat and simmer for 5 minutes. Put the tilapia in a baking dish, pour over the sauce and bake in the oven for 10-15 minutes. Serve garnished with basil.

Nutrition: calories: 281fat: 15.0g

protein: 23.0g carbs: 7.2g net carbs: 6.0g

fiber: 1.2g

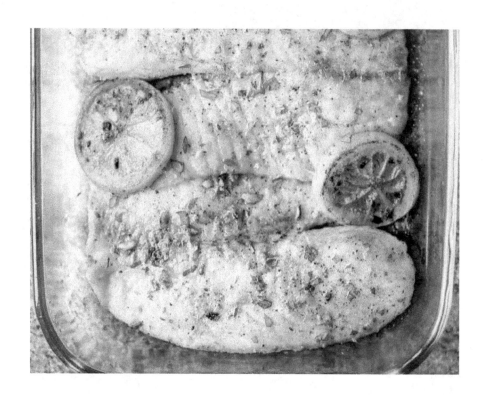

18.   Salmon Fillets with Broccoli

Preparation time: 10 minutes

Cooking time: 30 minutes

Servings: 2

Ingredients:

- 4 salmon fillets
- Salt and black pepper to taste
- 2tablespoons mayonnaise
- 2tablespoons fennel seeds, crushed
- ½ head broccoli, cut in florets
- 1red bell pepper, sliced
- 1tablespoon olive oil
- 2lemon wedges

Directions:

1. Brush the salmon with mayonnaise and season with salt and black pepper. Coat with fennel seeds, place in a lined baking dish and bake for 15 minutes at 370ºF (188ºC). Steam the broccoli and carrot for 3-4 minutes, or until tender, in a pot over medium heat.

2. Heat the olive oil in a saucepan and sauté the red bell pepper for 5 minutes. Stir in the broccoli and turn off the heat. Let the pan sit on the warm burner for 2-3 minutes. Serve with baked salmon garnished with lemon wedges.

Nutrition: calories: 564 fat: 36.8g protein: 53.9g carbs: 8.3g net carbs: 5.9g fiber: 2.4g

DESSERT

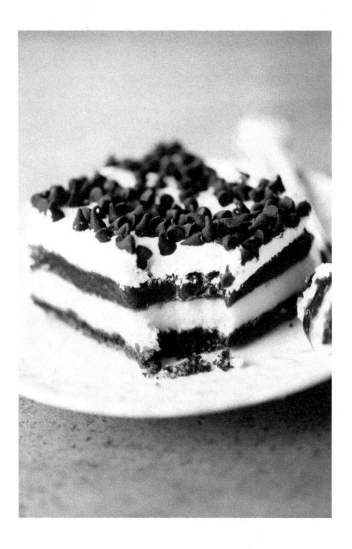

19. Chocolate, Berry, And Macadamia Layered Jars

Preparation Time: 10 minutes

Cooking Time: 3 hours

Serve: 8

Ingredients:

- 5 ounces dark chocolate, melted
- 1/2cup mixed berries, (fresh) – any berries you like
- 3/4 cup toasted macadamia nuts, chopped
- 7 ounces cream cheese
- 1/2cup heavy cream
- 1tsp. vanilla extract

Directions:

1. In a medium-sized bowl, whisk together the cream cheese, cream, and vanilla extract.

2. Spoon a small amount of melted chocolate into each jar or ramekin (only use half of the chocolate).

3. Place a few berries on top of the chocolate (use half of the berries).

4. Sprinkle some toasted macadamias onto the berries (use half of the nuts).

5. Spoon a dollop of the cream cheese mixture into the ramekin (use all of the cream cheese mixture).

6. Place another layer of chocolate, berries, and macadamia nuts on top of the cream cheese mixture.

7. Place the jars into the Crock Pot and pour enough hot water into the pot so that it reaches half way up the sides of the jars.

8. Place the lid onto the pot and set the temperature to LOW.

9. Cook for 6 hours.

10.   Remove the jars and leave them to cool and set on the bench for about 2hours before serving.

Nutrition: Calories 215, Fat 2, Carbs 1,

Protein 21

20. Salty-Sweet Almond Butter and Chocolate Sauce

Preparation Time: 10 minutes

Cooking Time: 4 hours

Serve: 8

Ingredients:

- 1cup almond butter
- 2ounces salted butter
- 1ounce dark chocolate
- 1/2tsp. sea salt
- Few drops of stevia

Directions:

1. Place the almond butter, butter, dark chocolate, sea salt, and stevia to the Crock Pot.

2. Place the lid onto the pot and set the temperature to LOW.

3. Cook for 4 hours, stirring every 30 minutes to combine the butter and chocolate as they melt.

4. Pour into a jar and leave to cool before storing in the fridge.

Nutrition: Calories 387, Fat 2, Carbs 1,

Protein 21

21. Coconut Squares With Blueberry Glaze

Preparation Time: 10 minutes

Cooking Time: 4 hours

Serve: 20

Ingredients:

- 2cups desiccated coconut
- 1ounce butter, melted
- 3 ounces cream cheese
- 1egg, lightly beaten
- 1/2tsp. baking powder
- 2tsp. vanilla extract
- 1cup frozen berries

Directions

1. In a large bowl, place the coconut, butter, cream cheese, egg, baking powder, and vanilla extract, beat with a wooden spoon until combined and smooth.

2. Grease a heat-proof dish (make sure it fits inside the Crock Pot) with butter.

3. Spread the coconut mixture into the dish.

4. Place the blueberries into a small bowl and defrost in the microwave until they resemble a thick sauce.

5. Spread the blueberries over the coconut mixture.

6. Place the dish into the crock pot and pour enough hot water into the pot so that it reaches half way up the dish.

7. Place the lid onto the pot and set the temperature to HIGH.

8. Cook for 3 hours.

9. Remove the dish from the pot and leave to cool on the bench before slicing into small squares.

Nutrition: Calories 365, Fat 1, Carbs 4,

Protein 26

22. Chocolate And Blackberry Cheesecake Sauce

Preparation Time: 10 minutes

Cooking Time: 4 hours

Serve: 20

Ingredients:

- 3/4 lb. cream cheese
- 1/2cup heavy cream
- 11/2ounces butter
- 3 ounces dark chocolate
- 1/2cup fresh blackberries, chopped
- 1tsp. vanilla extract

- Few drops of stevia (optional, depending on how sweet you prefer your sauce)

Directions:

1. Place the cream cheese, cream, butter, dark chocolate, blackberries, vanilla, and stevia into the Crock Pot.

2. Place the lid onto the pot and set the temperature to LOW.

3. Cook for 6 hours, stirring every 30 minutes to combine the butter and chocolate as it melts.

4. Pour into a jar and leave to cool before storing in the fridge.

5. Have a spoonful here and there to curb your sweet cravings! Or pour over Keto desserts or berries!

Nutrition: Calories 431, Fat 1, Carbs 2, Protein 12

23.   Peanut Butter Chocolate Cake

Preparation Time: 15 Minutes

Cooking Time: 3 Hours

Servings: 2

Ingredients:

- 15.25 oz devil eat cake mix
- 1cup water
- ½ cup melted salted butter
- 3 eggs
- 8 oz Package of Mini Reese's Peanut Butter Cups
- 1cup creamy peanut butter
- 3 caster sugar tsp
- Ten Reese's peanut *butter cups*

Directions:

1. In a large bowl, combine the cake mix, ice cream, butter, and eggs until smooth. Cut the mini peanut butter cups.

2. Melt butter in the pan and spread evenly.

3. Cover and cook on high for 2 hours.

4. Place the peanut butter in a small saucepan on the stove over medium heat. Stir until it is melted and smooth. Add the powdered sugar and beat to soften.

Nutrition: Cal 607, Carbs 57 g, Protein 13 g, Fat 39 g, Saturated Fat 13 g

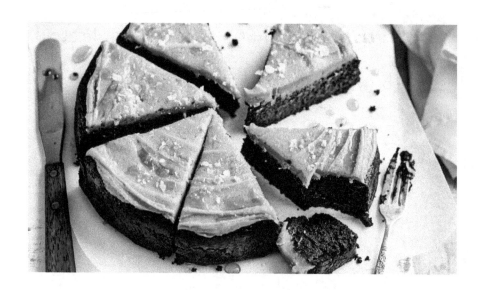

24. Crockpot Apple Pudding Cake

Preparation Time: 20 Minutes

Cooking Time: 5 minutes

Servings: 2

Ingredients

- 2 cups all-purpose flour

- 2/3 cup plus ¼ cup divided sugar

- 3 tsp of baking soda

- 1tsp salt

- ½ cup cold butter

- 1cup milk

- 4 apples, peeled and diced

- 1½ cup orange juice

- ½ cup honey or brown sugar

- 2 Tbsp melted butter

- 1tsp cinnamon

Directions:

1. Combine flour, 2/3 cup sugar, baking powder, and salt. Cut the butter until you have thick crumbs in the mixture.

2. Remove the milk from the crumbs until it becomes moist.

3. Grease the bottom and sides of a 4 or 5-liter slow cooker. Place the

dough at the bottom of the pot and spread it evenly.

4. Beat the orange juice, honey, butter, remaining sugar and cinnamon in a medium pan. Decorate the apples.

5. Place the jar opening with a clean cloth, place the lid. Prevents condensation on the cover from reaching the pot. Place the pan on top and cook until apples are tender for 2 to 3 hours.

Nutrition: Cal 405 Fat 9 g Saturated fat 3 g Carbs 79 g Fiber 2 g Sugar 63 g Protein 3 g

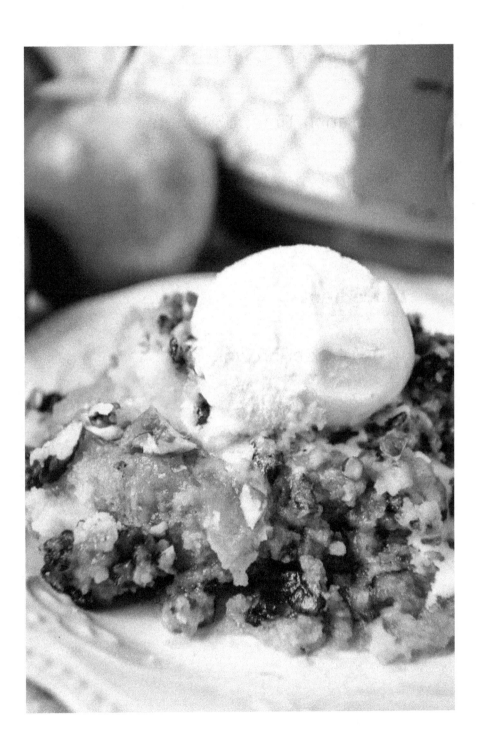

25. Brownie Cookies

Preparation Time: 15 Minutes

Cooking Time: 5 minutes

Servings: 2

Ingredients

- A box of brownie mix

- 2 eggs

- ¼ cup melted butter, ½ cup mini chocolate chips

- ½ c optional chopped nuts

- 8 slices of cookie dough or spoons filled with a bathtub

Directions:

1. If desired, combine your brownie mix with butter, eggs, chocolate chips, and nuts.

2. Sprinkle the inside of your slow cooker with a non-stick spray.

3. Place 8 slices of prepared cookie dough at the bottom.

4. Pour the brownie mixture into your slow cooker and smooth it evenly.

5. Put the lid on and cook for 2 hours.

Nutrition: 452 Cal, 21g fat, 7 g saturated fat, 59 g Carbs, 38 g sugar, 5 g protein

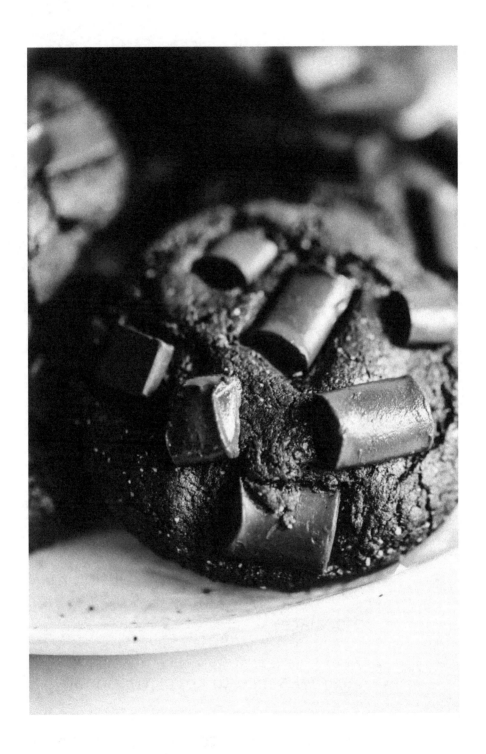

26. Chocolate Caramel Monkey Bread

Preparation Time: 10 Minutes

Cooking Time: 5 minutes

Servings: 2

Ingredients

- ½ Tbsp sugar

- ¼ tsp ground cinnamon

- 15 oz whey cookies

- 20 candies coated with milk chocolate

- caramel sauce to cover (optional)

- chocolate sauce to include (optional)

Directions:

1. Mix sugar and cinnamon and set aside.

2. Fill a jar with parchment paper, cover to the bottom.

3. Wrap 1buttermilk cookie dough around a chocolate candy to completely cover the candy and close the seam. Place the candy wrapped in cookies at the bottom of the jar, start in the middle of the pot and continue on the side.

4. Continue to wrap the candies and place them in the slow cooker, leaving about ½ inch between each. Repeat these steps with sweets

wrapped in the second layer of cookies. Sprinkle the rest of the sugar and cinnamon mixture over the dough.

5. Cover the pan and cook for 1hour 30 min. After cooking, remove the cover and allow it to cool slightly. Use the edges of the parchment paper to lift the monkey bread from the jar and move it onto a wire rack. Let cool for at least 10-15 min

6. Cut off the excess baking paper around the edge when you're ready to serve. Place the monkey bread in a shallow pan or bowl and sprinkle

with chocolate sauce and caramel sauce.

Nutrition: Cal 337k saturated fat 16g Carbs 44g Fiber 1g Sugar 12g Protein 5g

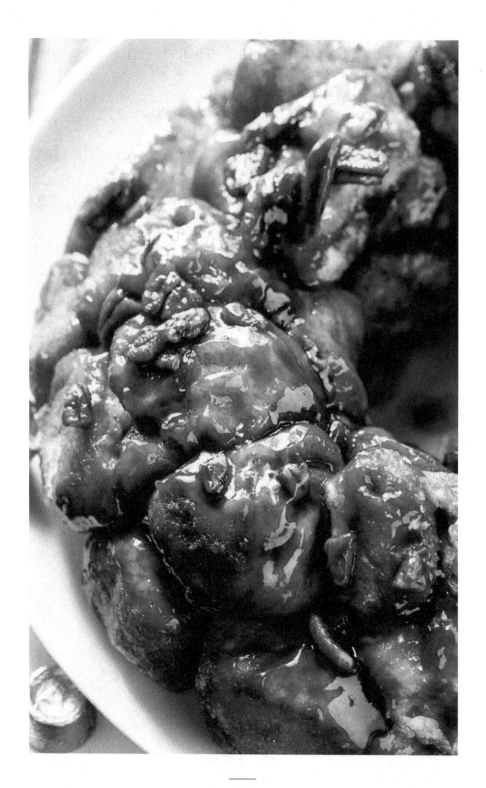

CPSIA information can be obtained
at www.ICGtesting.com
Printed in the USA
BVHW092304140621
609528BV00010B/1510